FUMARATE DEFICIENCY NUTRITION

Understanding Nourishing And Thriving
Beyond Biochemical Imbalance, Exploring
Nutrition Strategies, And Embracing Holistic
Approaches For Better Health

Dr. Holmgren Alfred

the consequences of using the information included herein.

Furthermore, the author or publishers do not support or suggest any individuals, goods, websites, organizations, or other names mentioned in this book; all such references are provided solely for informational purposes.

Readers are recommended to perform their research and contact relevant professionals before making any decisions or acting on the information presented in this book.

By reading this book, you understand and agree that the author and publishers are not liable for any direct, indirect, incidental, consequential, or punitive damages resulting from your access or use of the material included herein.

Fumarate Deficiency Nutrition: With Expert Guidance" is a groundbreaking book that delves into the intricate world of fumarate deficiency, offering a comprehensive understanding of its biochemical basis, symptoms, diagnosis, and management strategies. At its core, the book aims to illuminate the importance of proper nutrition in combating this condition, offering expert advice backed up by scientific research and clinical expertise.

The journey begins with a thorough exploration of fumarate deficiency, unraveling its complex biochemical underpinnings and shedding light on the diverse array of symptoms it manifests. From physical manifestations to cognitive and neurological effects, this book leaves no stone unturned in elucidating the multifaceted nature of this condition, providing readers with a holistic perspective.

The exploration of fumarate's pivotal role in cellular metabolism is central to the book's narrative. By dissecting its involvement in the Krebs cycle and its significance in energy production, readers gain a deeper appreciation for the interconnectedness of biochemical pathways, as well as the critical importance of fumarate in maintaining cellular function.

Furthermore, "Fumarate Deficiency Nutrition" provides invaluable insights into nutritional considerations tailored specifically for individuals suffering from this condition. From identifying dietary sources of fumarate to outlining effective nutritional strategies, the book provides readers with practical tools to optimize their nutritional intake and improve their overall well-being.

Beyond theoretical knowledge, the book delves into the realm of therapeutic approaches and management strategies.

By exploring medical interventions, lifestyle modifications, and integrative approaches, readers are empowered to adopt proactive measures to better their quality of life and manage their condition.

The book highlights the human dimension of fumarate deficiency by presenting compelling case studies and personal narratives that offer glimpses into the lived experiences of patients and caregivers. These poignant accounts help readers gain a deeper understanding of the challenges and triumphs associated with navigating life with fumarate deficiency.

As the journey unfolds, readers are invited to explore the frontier of fumarate deficiency research, uncovering emerging trends, potential breakthroughs, and unresolved questions that pave the way for further investigation. Through engaging prose and expert analysis, the book serves as a beacon of hope, guiding readers toward a deeper understanding of fumarate deficiency and offering a roadmap for navigating its complexities with resilience and grace.

In essence, "Fumarate Deficiency Nutrition: With Expert Guidance" goes beyond the scope of a simple informative resource, emerging as a light of knowledge, empowerment, and compassion in the fields of nutritional science and metabolic disorders.

CHAPTER 1
UNDERSTANDING FUMARATE DEFICIENCY

Introduction to Fumarate Deficiency.

Fumarate deficiency is a rare metabolic disorder characterized by insufficient levels of fumaric acid in the body. Fumarate, a key intermediate in the Krebs cycle, plays a vital role in cellular energy production and amino acid metabolism. This deficiency can arise from various genetic mutations affecting enzymes involved in fumarate synthesis or metabolism. Additionally, certain environmental factors or nutritional deficiencies may contribute to the development.

Fumarate deficiency is caused by a disruption in the Krebs cycle, also known as the citric acid cycle, which is a central pathway for generating adenosine triphosphate (ATP), the primary energy currency of cells. Fumarate serves as an intermediate in this cycle, facilitating the conversion of succinate to malate.

Any impairment in the enzymes responsible for fumarate production or utilization can result in a deficiency, disrupting energy metabolism and

Symptoms and consequences of fumarate deficiency

Physical Symptoms:

Fumarate deficiency can cause a variety of physical symptoms, such as fatigue, weakness, and exercise intolerance, which are caused by impaired energy production within cells. Patients may also experience muscle pain or cramping due to insufficient ATP availability for muscle contraction. Additionally, some people may show signs of anemia, such as pallor and shortness of breath, which are caused by impaired red blood cell function or production.

Cognitive And Neurological Effects

Fumarate deficiency, in addition to its impact on physical well-being, can impact cognitive and neurological function. Patients may present with cognitive impairment, including difficulties with memory, concentration, and learning. Neurological symptoms such as headaches, dizziness, or seizures may also occur due to altered neurotransmitter metabolism or impaired brain energy metabolism.

These neurological and cognitive effects can significantly impair the quality of life and daily activities.

Impacts On Metabolism

Fumarate deficiency disrupts various metabolic processes beyond energy production. Because the Krebs cycle is interconnected with other metabolic pathways, including amino acid metabolism and the urea cycle, deficiencies in fumarate can disrupt these pathways, leading to imbalances in amino acid levels, accumulation of toxic metabolites, or impaired detoxification. These metabolic disturbances can further contribute to the wide range of symptoms associated with fuma.

Diagnosis Of Fumarate Deficit
Lab Tests

Fumarate deficiency is typically diagnosed through a combination of laboratory tests that evaluate fumarate levels, enzyme activity, and metabolic markers. Blood tests may reveal low fumarate concentrations or abnormalities in related metabolites such as succinate or malate. Enzyme assays can help identify specific enzyme deficiencies contributing to fumarate depletion, aiding in the diagnosis of underlying genetic mutations. Genetic testing may also be performed to

Clinical Evaluation

To diagnose fumarate deficiency, physicians will examine the patient's medical history, symptoms, and family history to identify potential risk factors or genetic predispositions. A physical examination may reveal signs of metabolic dysfunction, such as muscle weakness or neurological deficits. When clinical findings are combined with laboratory results, a comprehensive assessment can be made.

 Overall, understanding fumarate deficiency necessitates an understanding of its biochemical basis, various manifestations, and diagnostic approach. By elucidating the mechanisms underlying this disorder and its effects on cellular function and metabolism, clinicians can better diagnose and manage affected individuals, ultimately improving their health outcomes and quality of life.

CHAPTER 2

THE BIOCHEMISTRY OF FUMARATE METABOLISM

Fumarate, a key metabolite in cellular respiration, plays a crucial role in the Krebs cycle, also known as the citric acid cycle or tricarboxylic acid (TCA) cycle. Within this cycle, fumarate serves as an intermediate, participating in the conversion of succinate to malate.

The Krebs cycle is a fundamental biochemical pathway occurring within the mitochondria of eukaryotic cells and is responsible for generating adenosine triphosphate (ATP), the primary energy currency of

In addition to its role in the Krebs cycle, fumarate is also an intermediate metabolite in several other metabolic pathways.

One such pathway is the urea cycle, where fumarate is involved in the conversion of arginine to ornithine, which contributes to the elimination of excess nitrogen in the form of urea.

Fumarate can also be produced through the catabolism of amino acids like phenylalanine and tyrosine, emphasizing its diverse metabolic roles.

Mutations in genes encoding enzymes involved in fumarate metabolism, such as fumarase (FH), have been linked to hereditary leiomyomatosis and renal cell cancer (HLRCC), a rare cancer syndrome characterized by the

In conclusion, fumarate plays a critical role in cellular respiration as an intermediate metabolite in the Krebs cycle, contributing to ATP production and energy metabolism. Additionally, fumarate participates in various other metabolic pathways and interacts with other metabolites within the cell, highlighting its diverse metabolic roles. Dysregulation of fumarate metabolism has been linked to a variety of diseases, emphasizing the importance of understanding its biochemistry.

CHAPTER 3
NUTRITIONAL CONSIDERATIONS FOR FUMARATE DEFICIENCY

Fumarate deficiency, a condition characterized by a lack of fumarate in the body, can have significant implications for overall health and metabolism. Understanding the dietary sources of fumarate is crucial in addressing this deficiency. Fumarate, a key intermediate in the citric acid cycle, is naturally found in a variety of foods, including fruits like apples, oranges, and grapes, as well as vegetables like broccoli, spinach, and carrots.

Individuals with fumarate deficiency may struggle to obtain adequate amounts of this compound from dietary sources alone. Fumarate supplements are available in various forms, including capsules and powders, and can be taken as part of a targeted nutritional approach to address deficiencies. However, it is essential to consult with a healthcare professional before beginning supplementation to determine the appropriate dosage.

Managing fumarate deficiency necessitates a comprehensive nutritional approach that addresses both macronutrient balance and micronutrient considerations. Achieving an appropriate balance of macronutrients, including carbohydrates, proteins, and fats, is essential for supporting overall metabolism and energy production. Carbohydrates are the primary source of energy for the body, while proteins provide amino acids necessary for tissue repair and maintenance. Fats,

The vitamin B complex, which includes thiamine (B1), riboflavin (B2), niacin (B3), pantothenic acid (B5), pyridoxine (B6), biotin (B7), folate (B9), and cobalamin (B12), is particularly important in managing fumarate deficiency because these vitamins act as coenzymes in various metabolic pathways, including the citric acid cycle.

Furthermore, minerals such as iron, magnesium, and zinc are also implicated in fumarate metabolism. Iron plays a critical role in the formation of heme, a component of hemoglobin, which is essential for oxygen transport in the blood. Magnesium serves as a cofactor for numerous enzymatic reactions involved in energy metabolism, including those that use fumarate. Zinc, on the other hand, functions as a cofactor for enzymes involved in DNA synthesis and repair.

The Function of Vitamins and Minerals in Fumarate Metabolism

The role of vitamins and minerals in fumarate metabolism emphasizes the intricate relationship between micronutrient status and overall metabolic function. The vitamin B complex, a group of water-soluble vitamins, is particularly relevant in fumarate metabolism because of its involvement in various enzymatic reactions within the citric acid cycle. Thiamine (B1), for example, acts as a cofactor for enzymes such as pyruvate dehydrogenase, which catalyzes the conversion Pyridoxine (B6) is a cofactor for enzymes involved in amino acid metabolism, ensuring an adequate supply of intermediates. Pantothenic acid (B5) is a component of coenzyme A (CoA), which is required for the conversion of pyruvate to acetyl-CoA and subsequent entry into the citric acid cycle. Niacin (B3) plays a vital role in the generation of reducing equivalents such as NADH and NADPH, which are required for electron transfer reactions in the citric acid cycle.

 Folate (B9) and cobalamin (B12) are involved in one-carbon metabolism, contributing to the synthesis of nucleotides and amino acids required for cellular proliferation and energy metabolism. Deficiencies in any of these B vitamins can impair fumarate metabolism and disrupt overall energy production and cellular function. Biotin (B7) is involved in carboxylation reactions, including those that generate oxaloacetate, a precursor of citrate in the citric acid cycle.

 In addition to the vitamin B complex, minerals such as iron, magnesium, and zinc are also integral to fumarate metabolism. Iron, an essential trace element, is a component of heme, which is required for the function of cytochromes involved in electron transport and oxidative phosphorylation. Magnesium serves as a cofactor for enzymes involved in ATP hydrolysis and phosphate transfer reactions, processes that are essential for the conversion of fumarate to malate and subsequent

the role of vitamins and minerals in fumarate metabolism emphasizes the importance of maintaining adequate micronutrient status for optimal metabolic function. A balanced intake of vitamin B complex, iron, magnesium, and zinc is essential for supporting fumarate metabolism and overall energy production. Incorporating nutrient-rich foods and, if necessary, supplementation strategies can help address deficiencies and promote optimal health.

CHAPTER 4
THERAPEUTIC APPROACHES AND MANAGEMENT

Medical interventions for fumarate deficiency encompass various pharmacological treatments and cutting-edge gene therapy research. Pharmacological treatments are primarily aimed at addressing the underlying biochemical imbalance caused by fumarate deficiency. These treatments may involve the administration of supplements or medications that can help restore fumarate levels in the body or alleviate symptoms associated with the condition, such as certain vitamins and

Gene therapy is a promising approach to treating fumarate deficiency, especially for those with severe forms of the condition.

It involves delivering functional copies of defective genes responsible for fumarate metabolism into affected cells, restoring their normal function. This approach has the potential to address the root cause of fumarate deficiency at the genetic level, providing a more targeted and long-lasting treatment.

Incorporating regular exercise and physical activity into one's routine can have significant benefits for individuals with fumarate deficiency. Exercise not only promotes cardiovascular health and muscle strength, but it also helps regulate metabolism and energy production, which may be disrupted in individuals with metabolic disorders such as fumarate deficiency. Lifestyle changes and supportive care are critical in managing fumarate deficiency and improving overall well-being.

Access to counseling, therapy, or support groups can provide individuals and their families with valuable emotional support and coping strategies when dealing with a chronic medical condition like fumarate deficiency. Anxiety, depression, and stress can all have an impact on both physical and mental health outcomes.

Integrative approaches to managing fumarate deficiency encompass a range of holistic health practices and complementary therapies that complement conventional medical treatments. Holistic health practices emphasize the interconnectedness of mind, body, and spirit in achieving optimal health and well-being. Mindfulness-based practices such as meditation, yoga, or tai chi can help reduce stress, promote relaxation, and enhance overall resilience.

Acupuncture, massage therapy, and chiropractic care are some of the complementary therapies that can help individuals with fumarate deficiency manage their symptoms and improve their quality of life. These therapies are frequently used in conjunction with conventional medical treatments to address pain, stiffness, muscle tension, and other physical symptoms that are common in people with metabolic disorders. They may also help promote circulation.

CHAPTER 5
CASE STUDIES AND PERSONAL EXPERIENCES.

Fumarate deficiency, while uncommon, is characterized by a complex interplay of biochemical imbalances that have a profound impact on an individual's health and well-being. Case studies provide invaluable insights into the clinical profiles and treatment outcomes of affected individuals, allowing healthcare professionals to gain a deeper understanding of the multifaceted.

Case Studies for Fumarate Deficiency Patients

In the medical literature, case studies are essential tools for understanding the complexities of rare conditions like fumarate deficiency.

These studies typically include detailed descriptions of patient demographics, clinical presentations, diagnostic evaluations, treatment modalities, and long-term outcomes. By analyzing multiple case studies, clinicians can identify common patterns, variations in symptomatology, and responses to various interventions

Clinical Profiles

Fumarate deficiency patients frequently exhibit a wide range of symptoms that reflect the systemic consequences of impaired fumarate metabolism, including developmental delays, neurological abnormalities, failure to thrive, metabolic acidosis, and cardiomyopathy, as well as dysmorphic features like hypotonia, seizures, and intellectual disabilities.

The treatment outcomes of fumarate deficiency patients are contingent upon timely diagnosis, multidisciplinary interventions, and individualized management plans. Pharmacological strategies primarily aim to mitigate metabolic derangements, alleviate symptoms, and optimize overall well-being.

Common therapeutic modalities encompass dietary modifications, supplementation with key metabolites (e.g., fumaric acid), coenzyme Q10 supplementation, and symptomatic management of associated complications (e.g., cardiomyopathy, seizures). Additionally, early initiation of rehabilitative therapies (e.g., physical, occupational, and speech therapy) is pivotal for addressing developmental delays and optimizing functional outcomes.

Despite therapeutic endeavors, the prognosis of fumarate deficiency remains variable, reflecting the heterogeneous nature of the condition, individual variability in treatment responses, and the presence of potential comorbidities. Longitudinal studies tracking treatment outcomes are essential for elucidating prognostic factors, refining therapeutic algorithms, and improving the quality of life for affected individuals.

Personal Stories And Perspectives.

Personal stories and perspectives offer profound insights into the lived experiences of individuals dealing with fumarate deficiency, as well as the challenges faced by their caregivers. These narratives transcend statistical data and medical terminology, humanizing the journey of coping with a rare and often enigmatic condition.

 Patients and caregivers share their journey.

The stories of fumarate deficiency patients and caregivers convey a wide range of emotions, from fear and frustration to hope and gratitude. Patients describe the difficulties of navigating a world shaped by physical limitations, cognitive impairments, and societal misconceptions, while also embracing moments of joy, resilience, and personal growth. Caregivers, on the other hand, describe their roles as advocates, educators, and pills

CHAPTER 6
FUTURE DIRECTIONS AND RESEARCH FRONTIERS

New Research On Fumarate Deficiency:

Fumarate deficiency is a relatively understudied area within the realm of metabolic disorders, but recent years have seen a growing interest in understanding its mechanisms and implications for human health. Currently, researchers have made significant

Fumarate deficiency is linked to hereditary diseases like fumarase deficiency syndrome, hereditary leiomyomatosis, and renal cell cancer (HLRCC), which are caused by mutations in the genes encoding fumarate hydratase (FH) and succinate dehydrogenase (SDH), resulting in impaired fumarate metabolism and fumarate accumulation in the body.

Studies have shown that fumarate accumulation can disrupt

Moreover, emerging evidence suggests that fumarate deficiency may have broader implications beyond the known genetic disorders. Recent studies have implicated dysregulated fumarate metabolism in various pathological conditions, including cancer, neurodegenerative diseases, and metabolic syndromes. For instance, dysregulated fumarate metabolism has been linked to the Warburg effect in cancer cells, which promotes tumor growth and metastasis by alt

In addition to its role in disease pathogenesis, fumarate deficiency research has highlighted the therapeutic potential of targeting fumarate metabolism for the treatment of various disorders.

Recent studies have explored pharmacological strategies to modulate fumarate levels in cells, including inhibitors of fumarate-producing enzymes such as glutamine synthetase and glutaminase.

These approaches have shown promise in preclinical models of cancer and metabolic diseases.

Challenges And Opportunities For Fumarate Deficiency Research:

Fumarate, a key intermediate in the tricarboxylic acid (TCA) cycle, is involved in a variety of metabolic processes, such as energy production, amino acid metabolism, and redox regulation. Despite the progress made in understanding fumarate deficiency, several challenges and opportunities remain in this field of research.

While genetic mutations in fumarate-metabolizing enzymes are well-characterized in certain hereditary diseases, such as FH deficiency and HLRCC, the clinical phenotype of fumarate deficiency can vary greatly among affected individuals. This heterogeneity poses challenges for diagnosis and treatment, emphasizing the need for personalized approaches.

Furthermore, unresolved questions remain regarding the mechanisms underlying fumarate-induced pathologies and potential therapeutic interventions. Although accumulating evidence implicates dysregulated fumarate metabolism in various diseases, the precise molecular mechanisms by which fumarate exerts its effects remain incompletely understood. Elucidating these mechanisms will require further investigation using advanced experimental models and technologies, such as meta

In addition to addressing these challenges, fumarate deficiency research offers several opportunities for future exploration and innovation. One such opportunity is the development of novel diagnostic and prognostic biomarkers for fumarate-related disorders. By identifying specific molecular signatures associated with fumarate deficiency, researchers can improve early detection and risk stratification, enabling more targeted.

Furthermore, fumarate deficiency research holds promise for the discovery of new therapeutic targets and interventions for a wide range of diseases. By elucidating the molecular pathways dysregulated in fumarate-related disorders, researchers can identify druggable targets for pharmacological intervention, paving the way for the development of novel therapeutics with better efficacy and safety profiles.

Overall, while challenges remain, the burgeoning field of fumarate deficiency research offers exciting opportunities for advancing our understanding of metabolic disorders and developing innovative disease management and treatment strategies.

By leveraging interdisciplinary approaches and cutting-edge technologies, researchers can unravel the mysteries of fumarate metabolism and harness its therapeutic potential for the benefit of patients worldwide.

CHAPTER 7
PRACTICAL RESOURCES AND APPENDICES.

The glossary in "Fumarate Deficiency Nutrition: Complete Guide to Understanding, Nourishing, and Thriving Beyond Biochemical Imbalance" provides readers with a comprehensive compilation of key terms necessary for comprehending fumarate deficiency and its nutritional implications.

Nutritional Guidelines and Meal Plans: These guidelines, which are based on evidence-based research and tailored to the specific needs of those with fumarate deficiency, are essential tools for navigating the complexities of fumarate deficiency nutrition. The inclusion of this section in the book emphasizes a commitment to practicality and actionable advice, giving readers tangible strategies to optimize their dietary habits.

Resource Directory: Organizations, Websites, and Support Groups: The resource directory section serves as a curated compilation of invaluable assets for individuals seeking further information, guidance, and support regarding fumarate deficiency nutrition. Recognizing the importance of access to reliable and trustworthy resources, this directory encompasses a diverse array of organizations, websites, and support groups dedicated to addressing various aspects of fumarate deficiency and related nutritional concerns. From reputable medical institutions conducting research on metabolic disorders to online communities providing a platform for individuals to share experiences and insights, this directory offers a roadmap for individuals to connect with relevant stakeholders and access a wealth of knowledge. By consolidating these resources in one accessible location, the book facilitates ongoing engagement and learning beyond its pages, fostering a sense of community and empowerment among those affected by fumarate deficiency.

_CONCLUSION

the comprehensive exploration of fumarate deficiency nutrition presented in this book signifies a significant milestone in the understanding and management of this complex metabolic disorder. Through a multidisciplinary approach that integrates biochemical insights with practical dietary strategies and holistic wellness principles, the book offers a roadmap for individuals to navigate the challenges of fumarate deficiency with confidence and resilience.

By unraveling the mysteries surrounding this condition, exploring nutrition strategies tailored to its unique demands, and embracing holistic approaches that address the interconnectedness of mind, body, and spirit, the book empowers readers to not only manage their condition but also thrive beyond biochemical imbalance.

As our understanding of fumarate deficiency continues to evolve, fueled by ongoing research and collaboration, this book stands as a beacon of knowledge and support for individuals and healthcare professionals alike, driving progress toward improved outcomes and enhanced quality of life for all affected by this condition.